Erectile Dysfunction

Prevent, Treat And Overcome
Erectile Dysfunction To
Give Your Sexual Life A Boost

By

Fhilcar Faunillan

1

Fhilcar Faunillan

Erectile Dysfunction

The information provided herein is stated to be truthful and consistent, in that any liability, in terms of inattention or otherwise, by any usage or abuse of any policies, processes, or directions contained within is the solitary and utter responsibility of the recipient reader. Under no circumstances will any legal responsibility or blame be held against the publisher for any reparation, damages, or monetary loss due to the information herein, either directly or indirectly.

Respective authors own all copyrights not held by the publisher.

The information herein is offered for informational purposes solely, and is universal as so. The presentation of the information is without contract or any type of guarantee assurance.

The trademarks that are used are without any consent, and the publication of the trademark is without permission or backing by the trademark owner. All trademarks and brands within this book are for clarifying purposes only and are the owned by the owners themselves, not affiliated with this document.

Table of Contents

INTRODUCTION

I want to thank you and congratulate you for downloading the book, *"Erectile Dysfunction: Prevent, Treat and Overcome Erectile Dysfunction to Give Your Sexual Life a Boost"*.

If you create a list of what guys are afraid of, not being able to get it up and perform in bed is surely there at the top. And this is no surprise since men get a sense of power and competence from being able to lead the bed game, get satisfaction from, and pleasure their partners. Failing to have an erection will hardly meet the goal of spending a sweaty time and its consistent occurrence will surely take its toll on a man not only emotionally and psychologically but socially as well. This is why erectile dysfunction is no picnic.

In some cases, the realization of having an Erectile Dysfunction or ED feels like a nightmare. Feelings of helplessness, emasculation, and powerlessness devour the man suffering from it and all these negative emotions will lead him to spiral down into behavior that could prove to be destructive for him and his partner.

Marital and sexual life specially suffers because the partners do not have an inkling on how to handle the case of having erectile dysfunction well. Instead of taking a proactive response about it, the tendency is that both the man and his partner passively reacts to what they think is a tragedy for their relationship.

In reality, yes, it is a concern but erectile dysfunction is not actually as horrible as it sounds. It is a condition whose permanence is not set in stone as it is curable. There is quite a significant level of embarrassment and terror associated with ED but this is only because of a lack of information about what this medical condition really entails.

Erectile Dysfunction

This book will not only expound more on the true definition of erectile dysfunction, it will also debunk the common myths people have mistakenly associated with it over the centuries in order to reassure you and give you a better understanding of how manageable erectile dysfunction is.

Furthermore, it will delve into the complications that you can expect to come hand in hand with erectile dysfunction so you will be better prepared for what is to come. Most importantly, this book contains tips to prevent erectile dysfunction and ensure that you will lead a healthier physical, emotional, and sexual life. Moreover, it discusses the multitude of ways to overcome erectile dysfunction – the therapies you can undergo, medications you can avail of, and other medical methods that can help you treat your condition.

This book is not only for men out there who are suffering from erectile dysfunction or fearing of experiencing one. This is also for women who have partners going through this condition. Remember, you can't just let your partner bear this problem all alone. If you want your sexual life to go back to what it was before or improve drastically, take matters into your hand and learn what you and your man can do in order to overcome erectile dysfunction.

Once again thank you for downloading this book and happy reading!

Chapter 1 - What Is Erectile Dysfunction?

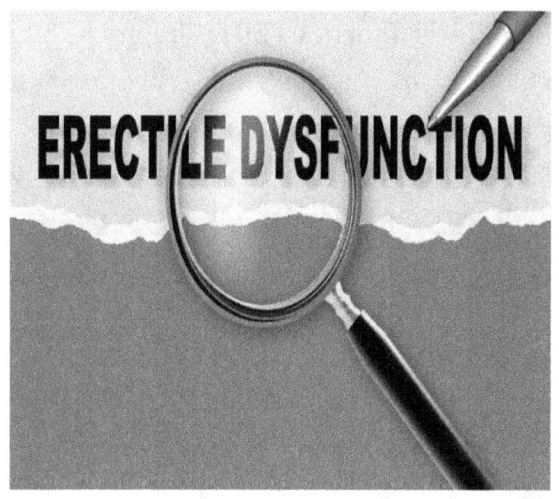

Failing to achieve an erection is an issue a man should not be embarrassed or concerned about. It happens to the best of you. Boys can have bad days, too! It could happen to anyone. Failing to attain an erection less than twenty percent of the time is in fact not that unusual and any form of treatment is hardly necessary. However, if it happens more than fifty percent of the time, it signifies that you have a major problem going by the name of erectile dysfunction in your hands.

Erectile dysfunction (ED) is defined as the inability to 'attain and maintain' an erection sufficient to allow satisfactory sexual performance. It is a serious issue as it can impact not only one's physical health but also affects it psychologically. Not to mention that ED will have a significant say on the quality of life (QoL) of both the sufferer and his partner. Mental well-being can deteriorate because of it and relationships will decline if it is not received well by the parties.

But what is the silver lining here is the fact that sufferers of ED can escape from the hell of unfulfilled sexual desires. And for men who fortunately have not had any problems with their erections, there are measures that they can take to give them a sense of guarantee that erectile dysfunction is not part of their near future.

Basically, being unable to attain or keep an erection adequate for sexual intercourse is the basic mark of ED but this problem can manifest itself in different ways. For some, their difficulties are transient and only appears occasionally. In this instance, the problem is not likely to be severe as we have already established that men will encounter troubles with their erections at some point.

In other cases, men have noticed that their dysfunction developed gradually but persistently. When chronic impotence happens, the cause is usually organic in form. This means that there are complications in bodily organs, systems, etc. that have contributed to the attainment of this condition. Diabetes for example, is among the many health conditions that can cause erectile dysfunction.

Additionally, there are other men whose erectile dysfunction advanced abruptly. However, they are still capable of developing early-morning erections and getting a stiffy when they are masturbating. In this scenario, the problem is probably psychological.

In the coming chapters, we are going to get into a more in-depth discussion on the underlying causes of erectile dysfunction. And each type of cause of ED has a corresponding ideal form of treatment. Unlike before when only a limited number of options are available for the affected man, science has now advanced to the point that there is a whole variety of treatments men can choose from as they take into consideration what they can afford, what caused their dysfunction, and what they are comfortable with.

Chapter 2 - The Truth Behind Erectile Dysfunction

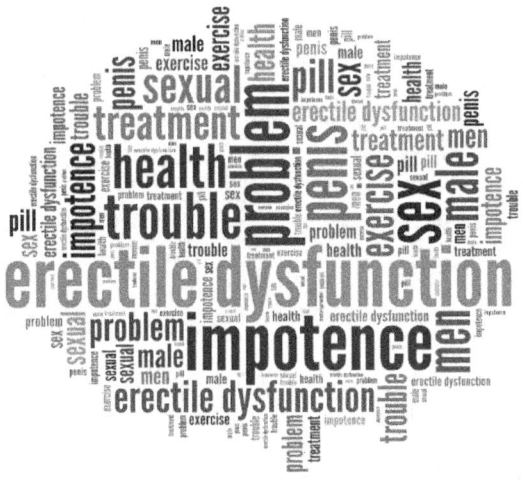

Since time immemorial, it has not been a secret that erectile dysfunction has been feared by men all over the globe. And part of that fear is brought about by a lack of awareness of what erectile dysfunction really is. Myths that do not hold grains of truth have been passed around, leading men to become paralyzed with anxiety. In this chapter, we are going to mention some of the most common misconceptions about erectile dysfunction that you should know the truth of.

1. Erectile Dysfunction is a result of masturbation.

This is a misconception that goes back to centuries and centuries ago. In a drive for sex in all its forms to be viewed as disgusting and unseemly but extreme religious purists, erectile dysfunction – known as impotence before – along with nervous disorders, blurred vision, logical deterioration, and reduction of strength, among others is claimed to be caused by masturbation. However, this is not true. There is no solid causal relationship between masturbation and the occurrence of erectile dysfunction.

2. It is a natural consequence of aging.

Yes, it is true that erectile dysfunction is more often seen in older men but this does not mean that it is a normal part of the aging process. Even our grandfathers still experience erection especially on early mornings. It should be considered as a medical problem that could ail any man regardless of the age since it *is* a medical problem.

3. Young men are safe from erectile dysfunction.

Since we have established that erectile dysfunction is in no way a given for men as they age, it is logical then to surmise that younger men are not exempted from suffering through erectile dysfunction. It can and will affect men of all ages if the contributing risk factors are present. Nowadays, this is becoming truer as we can observe that younger people are developing at a younger age diseases that can cause erectile dysfunction such as heart conditions, diabetes, and high-blood pressure among others.

4. **Erectile dysfunction only affects the man who is experiencing the condition.**

For the men who are going through ED and are reading this book, you can attest to the fact that erectile dysfunction truly does not affect just you but also your partners and anyone close who are privy to your situation. ED does not spare loved ones from this condition. A lover may feel rejected when you start detaching yourself from her or family members may end up extremely concerned if you choose a passive way to react to ED.

Part of the complications erectile dysfunction bring about in a man are the feelings of sadness, anxiety, frustration, anger, inadequacy, as well as feelings that could affect family and business relationships if they are not addressed properly.

5. Erectile dysfunction is all in a man's head.

In most cases, this misconception can be debunked. Various and diverse physical complications can lead to erectile dysfunction and they have nothing to do with his internal psychology. Contrary to what a lot of people think when they are asked about erectile dysfunction, men are suffering from it not because they are having issues with their sexuality or because they find their partners unattractive enough for an enjoyable time between the sheets. More often than not, these men might be going through other medical conditions that are causing ED such as injuries, pain conditions, and others.

However, it is also true that for some men, it is all in their head. Erectile dysfunction can stem from psychological issues that can affect their ability to achieve an erection and maintain it. Whether we realize it or not, just like women, men also feel anxious about how their bodies look and their ability to perform the sexual act. Post-traumatic stress disorder and other mental disorders can also be a risk factor for ED. A man can feel excited making up with his woman and when they are on the bed, one suddenly fears of something. It could be that hardening has started and when those thoughts of fear and anxiety flashes, the hardening halts and returns to its normal state. Perhaps many of you have experienced that and have felt frustrated. Not only you, your woman for sure have lost her excitement too and that feeling have been replaced by disgust and frustration.

6. Erectile dysfunction is permanent.

At the crux of a lot of men's and their partner's trouble with ED is the assumption that it is permanent. There is nothing more frustrating, power-draining, and discouraging than the assumption that the medical condition you are experiencing cannot be cured, that it will remain forever. This is where a lot of people are wrong when it comes to erectile dysfunction. It is not permanent. Therefore, any complications that you are experiencing because of it can be overcome.

Acknowledging that it is not will do a long way in improving your disposition and your relationship with your partner because if you treat it as just another temporary medical condition, you can avoid letting it destroy your confidence in yourself and reducing the quality of your relationship with your partner.

Chapter 3 - Why Can't I Get It Up?

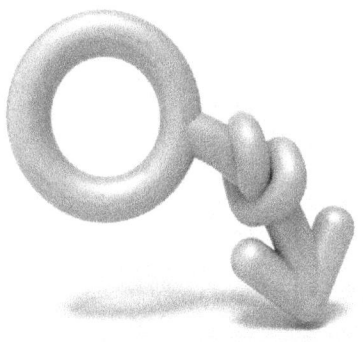

To better understand erectile dysfunction, let us delve first into the science of getting a boner. It is not as simple as men liking what they see or feel and responding accordingly. There is so much more to the erectile process than that. And knowing what it exactly entails would help us better handle it when erection fails.

The erectile process, taking place within one's body, is a complex one. It generally involves bodily systems including the central nervous system (CNS), peripheral nervous system (PNS) and a lot of other considerations such as blood flow and the penis itself. And what happens to the penis when a man is excited represents only a single step and it is not even the start of the tale.

When tactile, olfactory, auditory, and visual stimulation occurs (e.g. the sight of a woman undressing or a lover's hand on a man's erogenous zones), pathways in the brain are triggered. The brain then sends information down to nerve centers located at the base of the spine where you can find primary nerve fibers that are connected to the penis and are responsible for regulating blood flow during erections.

Moreover, sexual arousal leads to the release of chemicals from nerve endings found in the penis and these chemicals trigger a series of steps that cause the erection bodies of the penis to undergo muscle relaxation. These erection bodies have smooth muscles that control the blood flow into the penis. Relaxation of the smooth muscles would mean a dramatic increase in the blood flow, making the erection bodies to become rigid and full. The result is then the erection that we are familiar of. Erection is lost or the penis becomes flaccid when the chemicals that trigger muscle relaxation are no longer being produced.

In the processes I have discussed, any disruption in one or more of them could result to erectile dysfunction. Generally, we have two types of causes of ED: psychological and physical or organic causes.

For a lot of cases, erectile dysfunction is caused by organic ones or those related to problems with bodily organs. For some, the problem is associated with the quality of their mental health. However, the two causes are not mutually exclusive to each other. Psychological and organic reasons could play a life-altering combo.

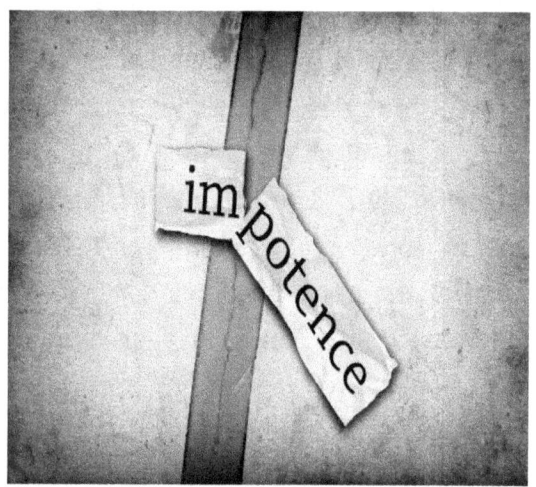

Organic Causes

As mentioned, physical causes of erectile dysfunction or impotency are much more common compared to psychological ones. Some of them are disease-related while others may pertain to injuries and other physical factors. In this section, I will go over the most common organic roots of ED.

1. *Diabetes*

>   When you think about what could probably cause erectile dysfunction, known diseases like diabetes do not really come into mind. In reality, they are actually risk factors for this medical condition. Diabetes is often overlooked because people may think abnormal blood sugar levels have nothing to do with your erection but they do. Diabetes can damage your nerves and blood vessels which are important to the achievement of an erection.

2. *Blood vessel diseases*

>   Blood vessel diseases are obvious underlying causes of erectile dysfunction. As vascular diseases

lead to the blocking of blood vessels, they are worrisome for they reduce the flow of blood towards the penis and making it hard to get an erection. Most common vascular diseases that can contribute to erectile dysfunction include atherosclerosis – a condition where there is a hardening of the arteries – high blood pressure, and high cholesterol.

3. *Neurological disorders*

As what I have mentioned earlier, your nervous system plays a great role in the erectile process. Without help from it, you will be unable to get an erection. Nerve and brain disorders that disrupt the transfer and delivery of information between your brain and penis can cause ED. Neurological disorders include multiple sclerosis, Alzheimer's disease, Parkinson's disease, and stroke.

4. *Kidney disease*

Kidney disease can cause a lot of changes in your body, changes which are not helpful for maintaining an erection. It can affect not just your hormones but also your nervous system and circulatory system. While you take in medication to remedy your kidney disorder, you must be aware that drug medication for kidney disease can also contribute to erectile dysfunction.

5. *Hormonal problems*

A man's sex drive and his ability to get an erection is fueled by testosterone and other hormones. Any imbalance to these hormones can lead to changes in his sex drive, making his body unable to initiate and complete the erectile process. Some reasons why hormones could go awry include tumors in the pituitary gland, prostate cancer treatment, and kidney disease, among others.

6. *Surgery*

There are cases when surgeries for cancers such as that of the prostate and bladder will damage tissues and nerves implicated in the achievement of an erection. When this happens, some men are lucky when the problem clears up after six to eighteen months. But in some cases, the damage is permanent and the man must then seek for treatment to address erectile dysfunction caused by the surgery.

7. *Venous leak*

Venous leak which can be caused by diseases and injuries can be a reason why you lose your erection. It is a condition when the blood that flows into your penis flows back out too quickly instead of staying, leading to the veins in your penis not constricting properly.

8. *Drug intake*

Drug abuse and intake of illegal substances will negatively impact your health and particular your ability to attain an erection. It is important to avoid substances such as alcohol, cocaine, marijuana, nicotine, and opiates not just so you can have a satisfying time in the bed but to also take care of your body.

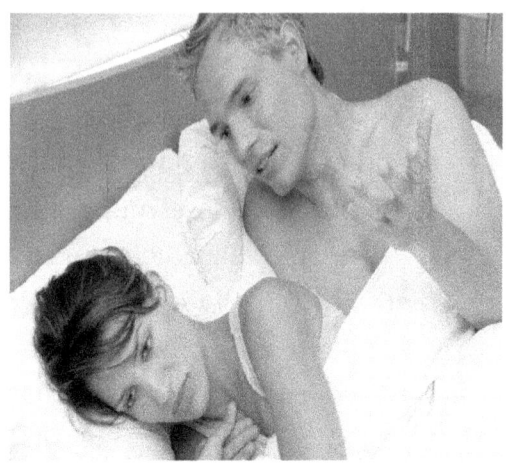

Psychological

At times, erectile dysfunction only happens in certain situations. While you can achieve an erection during masturbation or when you wake up, you probably are unable to do so when you are with your partner. In these cases, it is more likely that the reason of your erectile dysfunction is mainly psychological in nature.

For about fifteen percent of all cases of erectile dysfunction, psychological factors are mainly responsible for them. These psychological issues may be responses to existing physical ones or have originated from a history of sexual abuse and other kinds of trauma. The most common psychological reasons for ED though includes the following:

1. *Low self-esteem*

There are a lot of ways to hit a person's self-esteem. For men, one sure way to do so is attack their sexual capability and the quality of their performance. In cases when a man has experienced prior episodes of erectile dysfunction, this could result to him thinking that he is inadequate. Shame can wash over him at the thought that he would not be able to satisfy his partner. Aside from issues relating to sexual performance, there are a lot more factors that could contribute to the development of a

33

battered self-esteem. If left unaddressed, this psychological state, coupled with other mental and physical factors, could definitely bring about ED.

2. *Guilt*

ED can be exacerbated by previous experiences of not being able to achieve erection and pleasure a partner. Feelings of guilt can come out from such history.

3. *Stress*

We are all familiar with this. Stress is a major pain the ass as it is a risk factor for a lot of health diseases. Stress does not care about your sex life. It will invade every part of you if you do not know how to manage it.

Your situation at work, your financial status, the relationships that you have with other people, existence of any marital problems, etc. can overload your body with stress. The thing about stress is even though it is a purely psychological concept, it has a way of translating itself physically. And so you have clogged arteries, difficulty in breathing, fevers, and a weakened immune system, for example, because of it.

In the same way that stress affects your bodily systems, it could also impact those that are responsible for a healthy erection. And worse, it could cause one to have lack of interest in sex. Your body can become *'paralyzed'* and one feels tired and exhausted mentally which then can result to ED.

4. *Anxiety*

Let us face it. Men have insecurities, too. You might think it is only girls who are juggling issues about their bodies but guys actually hold some doubts about their competence, as well. And one of the most familiar matter that men actually fear is that they are not good enough in bed, that they do not know how to perform well. Society has set a convention that men are supposed to be those who need to take control, lead, and be masters of the sexual game and that expectation is a source of pressure on a man's part. Thinking that he is a failure at what is expected of him sexually could make the whole debacle an anxious one. It is common for men who are experiencing performance anxiety to not be able to reach or keep an erection and ending up unsuccessful in penetrating his partner, thus reinforcing his belief that he is no good in bed.

5. *Depression*

As what you will learn later in the succeeding chapter, depression can come off as a complication of erectile dysfunction but it can also be a precipitating factor that could lead to its development. Depression robs you out of your sexual drive and can affect the transport of signals from your brain to the systems in your body responsible for achieving a penile erection.

Chapter 4 - Complications

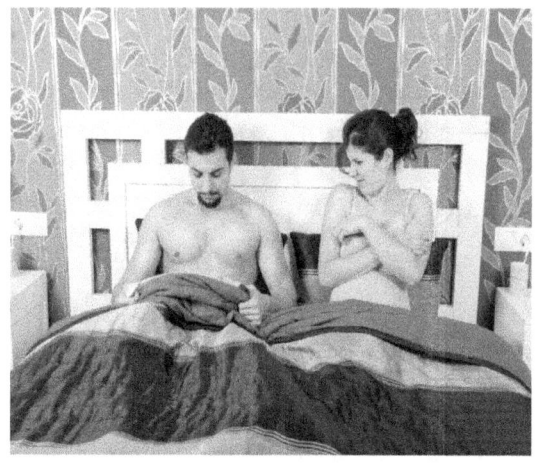

Getting it up is not the only problem you will be facing when you have erectile dysfunction. Together with the inability to achieve and maintain an erection fit for a satisfying time in bed are complications that can serve as hurdles for you and your relationships with other people. It is important to be aware of the other entailments of ED in order for you to know what to look out for and how they could possible affect your life. Only after becoming aware of these issues can you find it easy to solve them if ever they arise in your case.

Disappointing Sex Life

You saw this one coming – no pun intended – didn't you? A significant decrease in the quality of your sex life is the most palpable complication accompanying erectile dysfunction. As much as it sucks, sex life will seriously take a hit and will end up less fulfilling. And what is worse, your partner will also suffer as a result of the unsatisfactory situation. After all, it is such a shame to just stick with oral sex forever, right?

Unlike other implications of erectile dysfunction, you can't do too much about the issue of substandard sex because until you cure yourself of ED, it is just hard to find a way around it. Unless, of course, you are the kind of guy who is a genius in bed and can think of creative and highly gratifying ways to enjoy sex even without the participation of your penis. But the sad truth is, not everyone is good at the art of lovemaking and so, finding a way to get over this issue while you are still facing the problem of having ED can end up to be frustratingly tricky. But do not let all my talk get you down. After all, you are reading this book to find solutions and boost your sex life and you will discover just that on later parts of this book. In time, you will be again leading an exciting and fulfilling sex life with your partner (or various ones).

Marital Issues

Sex should not be just what is at the core of any intimate marital relationship; but admittedly, it is an important one. Backing this, statistics say that a considerable number of failed marriages have direct and indirect connections to erectile dysfunction. This may be attributed to how values that should be nurtured to make a relationship continue and grow such as trust, openness, intimacy, and closeness are affected by how a couple mistakenly handles the problem of ED and the corresponding failure to start any satisfactory sexual sessions. For example, a guy, out of low self-esteem and embarrassment, could distance himself and withdraw emotionally. His partner may interpret this move as a lack of interest in his part and letting this assumption bleed into her own self-esteem and feelings of attractiveness.

Moreover, depressed men, especially during times when they have hit rock bottom, could neglect his relationship with his partner while women may fail to understand men's predicament. For other women out there, the mistaken belief that ED is not curable may get them thinking that they would not ever be sexually satisfied ever again. In all these scenarios, the relationship suffers and could lead to dissention and dissolution.

Depression

Sex is a basic physiological need and this makes it a major part of human lives. For men, it can be a source of their power and sense of efficacy. Most, if not all, consider their sexual ability as a way of measuring their masculinity. Failing to perform, therefore, can emasculate them. With the sense of emasculation comes the feelings of frustration, worthlessness, and embarrassment at the reduced sexual ability and all of these could be contributing factors to the development of depression.

Studies have actually shown that erectile dysfunction has high comorbidity with depression and anger. Not only that, those suffering from ED reported to have high levels of anxious symptoms and psychological distress and reduced quality of life as well as that of compromised occupational and social functioning.

Results of researchers are not a surprise as it is very easy to understand why men who have ED end up being depressed given that sex and the ability to exercise it plays major roles in how they see themselves. Moreover, as there is a sense of responsibility in taking charge of lovemaking and pleasuring their partner, it is definitely a blow to their psyche that they can't meet those expectations.

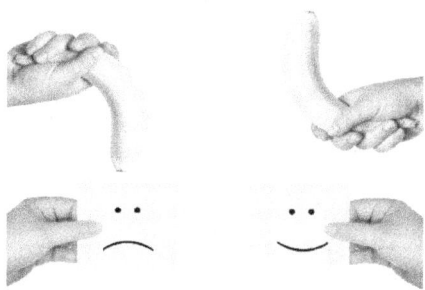

Low Self-Esteem

In contrast to other kinds of failure, failing to achieve and maintain an erection is in a whole another level. As a guy, failing an exam is less than a blip on your "I-care" radar. You can always study for the next one, ace it, and eradicate any negative insinuations on your intelligence. Erectile dysfunction, on the other hand, can make you feel less of a man and this feeling is not so easy to overcome as it is the ego that is directly threatened. A man's pride, despite seeming to be invulnerable, is actually really fragile given certain situations. ED is a bomb that is a sure-fire way of blowing and breaking a man's self-esteem into a million pieces. Those who suffer from it will feel extremely embarrassed and insufficient and these feelings, along with others, can create a caustic brew that could lead to greater issues (e.g. depression.)

Erectile Dysfunction

Yes, a diminished self-esteem happens when one suffers through ED. Yes, depression can happen. Yes, a psyche continually feeling embarrassed could develop. But do you know what *should* happen? Nothing. Yep. Nothing. I know that this may be very easy for me to say but absolutely nothing should happen. Guys should not feel like their worth as a person has decreased just because they are having this problem. It is just another medical problem. Fevers, measles, diarrhea are medical ailments but you do not see anyone beating themselves up over the fact that they have somehow contracted those issues.

Chapter 5 - Prevention

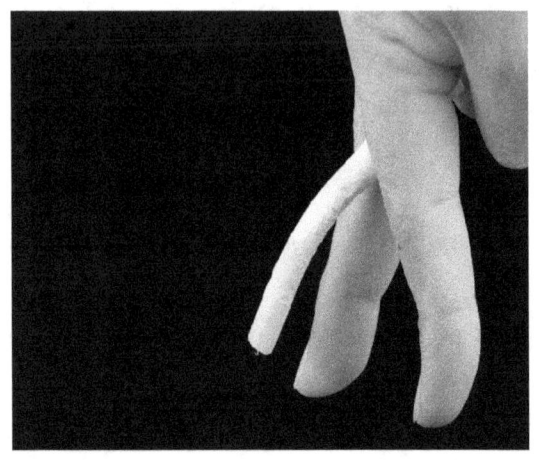

Now that we have learned as much as we could about erectile dysfunction, let us move on to how you can proceed to overcoming it. But first, for those who are reading this book and are not yet experiencing ED, this section is for you. Below are ways to prevent the development of erectile dysfunction. Following these steps will greatly help you avoid ED. But for men who is now going through erectile dysfunction, preventive measures for ED are not something that you should dismiss because as effective as they are in fighting against the attainment of ED, they are also good methods to take in abetting you improve your condition. For others, especially for minor cases of dysfunction, embracing preventative steps can actually relieve you of your condition depending on how faithful you are to those steps.

Lead a healthy lifestyle

Lifestyle can absolutely play a role in the development of erectile dysfunction. Smoking too much, being overweight, and leading a sedentary lifestyle, among others can affect good blood flow which is the key to achieving and maintaining erections. Leading a healthy lifestyle does not just ensure that you the risk of having ED is considerably reduced, it also helps you avoid contracting other serious health problems like cancer, heart conditions, hypertension, etc.

1. ***Stop smoking.***

    Smoking makes it more possible for a person to develop atherosclerosis, a condition that involves the hardening of the arteries resulting to a reduction in the blood flow throughout one's body not excluding the penis and thus affecting a man's capability of gaining an erection.

2. ***Watch your weight.***

    Being overweight can complicate your health in a lot of different ways. For one, it increases the risk of getting vascular diseases that could block your blood vessels and affect the flow of blood to and within your penis. The probability of developing diabetes is also heightened.

3. *Veer away from sedentary lifestyle.*

A sedentary lifestyle is often the fundamental root of many health problems. Being a couch potato and not moving even a finger because of laziness can affect the health in detrimental ways. Embracing this kind of lifestyle makes it easier for people to end up overweight because exercise will never be part of their schedule. And too much fat in the body could impact blood circulation into the penis, making it unable to get erect.

4. *Watch what you are eating.*

Studies have implied that eating foods that could contribute to the attainment of heart attacks brought about by restricted blood flow in the coronary arteries could likewise hamper the blood flow to and within a man's penis. And we know that blood flow is one of the keys of having an erection.

It is therefore important to watch what you eat as more or less of a certain food type could cause the development of ED. Partaking in very few vegetables and fruits and a lot of fried, processed, and fatty foods can reduce your body's blood circulation.

You should take note not to devour particular those rich in cholesterol since a high level of cholesterol in the body will impair the blood vessels including those that bring blood to your penis. To be sure, you can go to your doctor from time to time and let him check your cholesterol levels to find out if you are safe.

Just think of it this way: what is probably bad for your general health is also bad for your penis as it is a part of your body.

5. *Regulate alcohol-intake*

Men can attest to the fact that a little bit of alcohol can up their sexual game. It can improve sexual performance but this beneficial effect is extremely short-termed. There is nothing to fuss on if you exercise modicum intake of alcohol as it would not do any permanent bodily damage. Abusing alcohol, on the other hand, is another story. Too much alcohol can result to nerve damage and liver problems that can affect the erectile process.

Manage your medical conditions

The main idea behind managing your physical medical conditions is so you can eliminate some of the risk factors that could lead you to develop an erectile dysfunction. Do not let any chronic medical diseases go untreated and neglected.

Make sure to regulate your blood pressure and manage your cholesterol levels through proper diet, exercise, and necessary medication to avoid any damage and blockage to your blood vessels.

If you have diabetes, it is very much recommended to address that and take the proper treatment so this disease would not cause too much damage on your nerves and cause ED.

Bear in mind to do regular physical check-ups in order to have a better understanding of the state of your body.

An annual regular physical examination will do and it will go a long way to help you prepare and prevent any serious medical issues.

Take mental health into consideration

You know by now the role of stress, anxiety and other mental states have on the attainment of erectile dysfunction. So, it is a very good prevention method to take your mental health into consideration. Mental issues can create a vicious cycle and so they must be addressed accordingly. For example, if you are feeling extremely anxious, this could contribute to you failing to get an erection. And once that failure happens, you end up beating yourself up.

Once you have determined that you are dealing with a certain mental issue, try to think about how you can remedy it. If, for an instance, you are feeling overwhelmed by stressful events around you, find ways to relieve yourself of that stress.

If, on the other hand, you believe that what you are going through is much more serious and chronic, do not be ashamed and do not hesitate to ask for professional help.

Bottom line is, do not think that you have to always be strong. Learn to admit needing help from other people. Mental issues could be hard to deal with so don't be too much of a scaredy-cat to ask for some extra hands.

Talk to your partner

This is an important preventative measure that is often dismissed by a lot of men and couples out there. Talking, as easy it is to do, is avoided by coupes with or without problems. Maybe they find that there is too much work involved or it is too intimate but it is necessary for any relationship to work. And how does it help prevent ED? Well, it helps alleviate any mental complications that are starting to rise.

For men with performance anxieties, keeping an open communication with their partners will be a tool to relieve that worry. If you think that your skills in bed are not sufficient for satisfactory play, man up and tell your partner. It gives you both the chance to discuss and affirm or debunk your claim. That way, you will certainly know if your fears have basis and if ever it is true, you can know what you are doing wrong. That way, you know what to work on and you can build your confidence from there.

Talking to a person that you have an intimate connection with will also go a long way in discharging any stress that might have accumulated from other aspects of your life. Even if the problem is your relationship itself and it is what is making you stressed nowadays, talking will help resolve any issue that you and your partner might be experiencing.

Chapter 6 - Starting The Healing Process

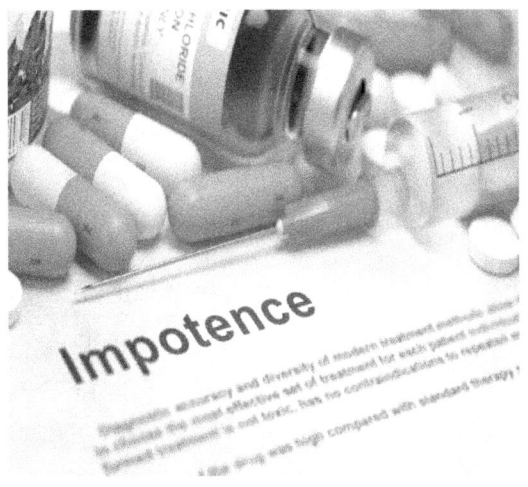

To start, when it has come to your attention that you are suffering from erectile dysfunction, it is recommended to come see a doctor or general practitioner so you can be properly diagnosed. In this section, we are going to go into what you can expect during your appointment with your doctor.

To start off, it would be better if you prepare yourself for your session. For one, when you are making your appointment, make sure to ask your doctor what you need to do in advance. He might like you to avoid eating certain types of food or veer away from certain behaviors before your appointment.

And to make your appointment go smoothly, you can prepare beforehand by writing down the symptoms that you have had so there would not be a chance that you missed reporting something to your doctor. You can also include any personal information relevant to your condition such as major life events and stresses, what medications, supplements, and vitamins you have taken, and any questions you might have for your doctor.

Some of the questions you could ask your doctor could include the following:

Erectile Dysfunction

1. What is the cause of my erectile problems?

2. Will my erectile dysfunction be permanent or temporary?

3. What tests do I need to take?

4. What treatment do you suggest I take?

5. Can you discuss other available treatment methods for erectile dysfunction?

6. Do I need to see a specialist?

7. What is the cost of treating erectile dysfunction?

8. Will medication be prescribed?

In turn, your doctor will be asking you questions. When you bring up the issue of erectile dysfunction, the following are some of the inquiries that you should expect and answer:

1. Do you have other sexual problems?

2. What changes have you experienced when it comes to your sexual desire?

3. Do you get erections when you masturbate?

4. Do you get erections when you wake up?

5. Do you get erections while you are with your partner?

6. Are you and your sexual partner experiencing any problems with your relationship?

7. Does your partner have sexual concerns?

8. Do you have other health problems or chronic medical conditions?

9. Are you under stress?

10. Are you anxious or depressed?

11. Are you currently diagnosed with a mental health condition? If yes, do you take any medication for that or engage in psychological therapy?

12. When did you first notice being unable to achieve and maintain an erection?

13. Do problems with your erection occur just sometimes, often, or all the time?

14. Are you taking any medications right now including supplements and remedies?

15. Do you smoke? How often?

16. Do you drink alcohol? How often and how much?

17. Do you use illegal drugs?

18. Did you notice any situation wherein your erectile dysfunction symptoms improved?

19. Did you notice any situation wherein your erectile dysfunction symptoms worsened?

In most cases of men who are suffering from erectile dysfunction, their appointment with their doctors only require a physical exam and for questions regarding medical history to be answered before the doctor is able to diagnose that the man is indeed experiencing ED and recommend a method of treatment. However, depending on what your health conditions have revealed, further tests may need to be performed which includes the following:

1. ***Blood tests***

    Blood tests will help the doctor determine if you have diabetes, heart problems, and issues with your hormones, among other health conditions. Knowing your medical issues will go a long way in determining the proper treatment method for your erectile dysfunction.

2. ***Physical exam***

    Expect that in physical examinations, your penis will be under examination as the doctor checks it along with your testicles for any sign of abnormalities.

3. ***Urinalysis***

Urinalysis serves the same purpose of blood tests. They are also utilized to find any diseases such as diabetes.

4. *Lipid profile*

This particular test will measure the amount of fats that you have in your body and that includes how much cholesterol you have. It is important to know your cholesterol level since a high level of it may signify that you have atherosclerosis.

5. *Thyroid function test*

Hormones produced from your thyroid abet in regulating the levels of your sex hormones. When there is a problem with your thyroid, it could cause a deficiency in thyroid hormones, affecting the level of sex hormones in your body.

6. *Duplex ultrasound*

Duplex ultrasound is utilized in handling cases of men with erectile dysfunction to check blood flow and any sign of tissue scarring, venous leak, and atherosclerosis. It is usually done while the penis is rigid – with the help of a drug that stimulates erection being injected into the penis – and while it is flaccid.

7. *Penile biothesiometry*

This kind of test requires the usage of an electromagnetic vibration that helps in figuring out proper functioning and sensitivity of nerves. When there is a decrease in sensitivity compared to what is average, this may mean that is the man has a nerve damage impeding the successful achievement of an erection.

8. *Bulbocavernosus reflex*

In this test, the objective is to determine a man's nerve sensation in his penis. What a doctor does is squeeze the head of the penis, expecting that by that action, the rectum will immediately contract. If there is a problem with nerve functioning, there will be a delay in the contract of the rectum or the absence of a response altogether.

9. *Arteriography*

This test is necessary for men with ED who are potential candidates for vascular reconstructive surgery. It is done by injecting a dye into the artery assumed to be damaged and then an X-ray is taken.

10. *Overnight erection tests*

Overnight erections tests are utilized to determine whether the cause of your erectile dysfunction is physical or psychological in nature. In some cases, men have reported to not being able to attain erections at all when in fact, during their sleep, their penis have stiffened without them remembering.

This test involves the issue of a device that will be wrapped around a man's penis before he goes to bed. This device will then measure the frequency and intensity of erections that happen overnight.

11. *Psychological exam*

Your doctor might also ask you questions that could tell him whether or not you are suffering through symptoms of mental health issues that could be the underlying reason for your erectile dysfunction.

Chapter 7 - Overcoming Erectile Dysfunction

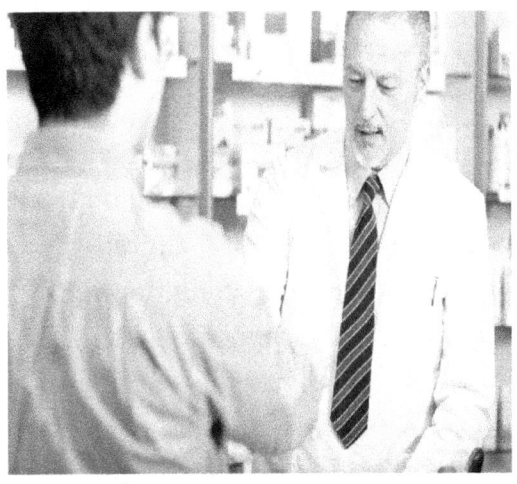

If you have met with your doctor and had him diagnose you, it is most likely that he has also suggested the best treatment method for your situation. Depending on the cause, ideal treatment might vary. But for those who have not had the chance to see their doctors or felt like they do not need one right now because they are fairly certain that they do have ED, this chapter is where the ways to overcome

ED will be reviewed. You can go over these options and think about which will suit you – your budget, partner, etc – best.

Lifestyle Change

A change in lifestyle is not also embraced to prevent erectile dysfunction but to also treat it. This is the most natural way you can respond to your condition and it is fairly inexpensive and easier to achieve compared to other kinds of treatment. The following are some of the lifestyle changes that you can commit to in order to relieve erectile dysfunction:

1. Exercise regularly.

2. Quit smoking.

3. Eat healthier foods.

4. Avoid high-fat foods.

5. Maintain a normal weight.

Oral medications

For about seventy-five percent of men in the general population who try them out to treat the organic causes of erectile dysfunction, oral medications have been proven to be effective. Available as prescription medicines, oral medications for ED include sildenafil (Viagra), vardenafil (Levitra), and tadalafil (Cialis).

What makes these medications effective is that they augment the effects of nitric oxide, a natural chemical produced by the body that relaxes the muscles in your penis to allow more blood to flow in so that you can get an erection in response to sexual stimulation.

Viagra, in particular, works by dilating the blood vessels and improving the blood circulation in the penis. It should be taken an hour on an empty stomach before sex and can work for roughly four hours. It comes in doses of 25 mg., 50 mg., -- the average suggested dosage – and 100 mg.

Just remember that Viagra, unlike what a lot of people think, does not heighten a man's sexual desire. There must be arousal for it to be effective.

Like Viagra, Levitra also abets in increasing the blood flow to the penis and making men get an erection during sex. It must also be taken 1 hour before sex. Available in doses of 2.5 mg., 5 mg., 10 mg., and 20 mg., Levitra should not be taken more than once a day.

Cialis differs from the other two drugs in the matter of effect longevity. Unlike Viagra and Levitra that only works for four hours, the effects of Cialis can last up to thirty-six hours. But like the others, it also helps by increasing the blood flow to the penis when the man is sexually aroused, letting him achieve an erection satisfactory for sex. Even for those suffering from moderate and severe erectile dysfunction, Cialis has been clinically proven to bring improvement.

There are drawbacks, though, to using Cialis. The most common side effects that it brings include an upset stomach, headaches, muscle aches, and back pain. But do not worry, these side effects go away a few hours after taking Cialis.

Cialis comes in 5 mg., 10 mg., -- the suggested starting dose – and 20 mg. tablets. In contrast to Viagra, since Cialis is not affected by your intake of high-fat foods and foods in general, you do not need to have an empty stomach before you can take it.

However, it must be noted that these tablets do not automatically trigger an erection by themselves as sexual stimulation is still necessary beforehand to release the body's nitric oxide from your penile nerves. What they do is strengthen the body's response to sexual stimulation to allow men with ED to function normally.

Sex therapy

For men suffering from ED whose roots are primarily psychological, sex therapy is the best option for you. A short-term kind of counselling, sex therapies consist of five to twenty sessions with a sex therapist who will help you deal with mental issues that might be driving factors behind your erectile dysfunction. Length of sexy therapy sessions depends on the therapists or any agreement you will have with him or her. Usually, they can last up to an hour and takes place every week.

Expect that therapists might assign you tasks to do at home including reading materials about sexuality, engaging in exercises that are intended to eradicate the pressure to perform brilliantly during sexual activities, and together with your partner, practicing sexual communication skills.

Sex therapy works for those who can achieve an erection while asleep and are in relatively good health. It is also ideal for men whose ED are caused by anxiety and stress brought about by work, finances, social relationships, and poor sexual relationships. The effectiveness of sex therapy also heightens when the man suffering from ED has his partner with him during the sessions. Having the partner in the therapy makes it easier and faster for problem resolution.

If you choose to go for sex therapy, remember to consistently attend your sessions. It would not work if you drop out of the psychological treatment after only one session.

Penile Surgery

Penile surgery is the road to take when the underlying factor behind erectile dysfunction is physical in nature. It is done to reconstruct the arteries within the penis in order to increase the flow of blood, thus, helping the achievement of an erection; implant a penile prosthetic device; or block off veins that permit blood to leave the penis so it can maintain an erection.

Depending on the goal that you want to meet, you can choose to undergo either implantation of a prosthetic device or vascular reconstructive surgery.

1. *Penile prosthesis*

Before, penile prosthesis was the only treatment method seen to be effective in curing erectile dysfunction with an organic cause. But now, it is the last option to be considered as it requires surgery. Before resorting to surgical options, doctors prefer to go for and try nonsurgical options. This does not imply, however, that implantation of penile prosthetics is an unreliable method since over the years, it has proven its effectiveness.

It is of course a given that your doctor will discuss any benefits and risks related to penile implant.

To give you a better idea of penile implant, at this point, let us discuss what exactly a penile prosthesis is.

Penile prosthesis is a device that can be either bendable (malleable) or inflatable, the former of which is the simplest kind of prosthesis.

Malleable prosthesis consists of two matching cyliners that doctor surgically implants within the erection chambers of a penis. If you go for this certain type of penile implant, your penis will end up always semi-rigid and all you have to do to initiate sex is lift and manually adjust the position of your penis.

Some of the advantages of opting for malleable implants include the simple surgery it requires and its relatively few complications. Furthermore, it is the least expensive implant there is and more importantly, it is highly effective with an eighty percent success rate.

The drawbacks that you have to bear, though, if this is your choice include the fact that implanting malleable rods within your penis would require surgery and the difficulty to conceal your penis since it would always be in a semi-rigid state. This means that you will practically have a constant erection. You also run the risk of destroying the natural erectile process and altering erection bodies once the device has been implanted. And just a note, malleable implants would not increase the width of your penis.

Inflatable implants, on the other hand, have its own appeal. They are made of two cylinders that are inserted into your penis through surgery, a pump which will be placed in your scrotum, and a reservoir of fluid that will be situated either in a different reservoir located beneath the tissue of your lower abdomen or within the two cylinders.

The inflatable implants work when you squeeze the pump positioned within the scrotum, the pumping action inflating the cylinders. The pump achieves this by moving the fluid found in the reservoir towards the cylinders that have been implanted in the penis. What creates an erection is the inflation of these cylinders. To make the penis return to its flaccid state, all you have to do is press a deflation valve which you can find at the base of the pump. This will trigger the fluid to return to the reservoir and will deflate the penis.

Inflatable implants can work up to ten years before you would need to replace it. The good news is that most companies who sell inflatable implant offer lifetime warranties for its components.

What is enticing about getting inflatable implant is that it simulates the natural erectile process of the penis becoming rigid and flaccid. Additionally, unlike malleable implants, guys can control the state of your erection and you would not get stressed over trying to conceal your boner. And some of you may really like this perk but inflatable implants can also increase the width of your penis.

On the flip side, its complications include risks of infection and the high probability that the device will malfunction. Given the process that it takes for inflatable implants to work, mechanical failure is to be expected. In addition, it is also the most expensive kind of implant and like malleable implants, it can injure your erection bodies.

Now that we have gone over both kinds of penile prosthesis, you might wonder if the prosthesis is noticeable enough to bring you embarrassment. Do not fret. Those who went through implantation can pinpoint the tiny scar involved in the surgery but other people can't. If you have within your penis inflatable implants, others would not be able to tell that you have them. So, being in a public restroom or locker room with other guys would not be a nightmare for you. As for malleable implants, that is obviously different. You know what to expect if you walk around naked while you have on your malleable implants. They will totally wonder why you are constantly erect.

With regards to your sex life after you have had prosthesis surgically implanted within your penis, there is nothing to be extremely concerned about. Upon erection of your penis, the prosthesis will make it thick and rigid just like natural erections. What is more, it will not change your capability of reaching an orgasm nor will it alter the sensations that you feel on the skin of your penis. Rest assured that ejaculation will not be impacted. In general, prosthesis are suitable for pleasurable sexual intercourse and can satisfy both you and your partner.

2. *Vascular reconstructive surgery*

This type of surgical treatment is done for the purpose of rebuilding the arteries within the penis to facilitate increase in blood flow and making it possible for the man to achieve and maintain an erection. It can also be administered in a way that it will block off the veins within the penis. By doing so, blood will stay within the penis so it can remain erect.

The greatest advantage vascular reconstructive surgery has over penile prosthetic implantation is that, in case of success, it can restore your natural erection. You also do not have to worry about the cosmetic appearance of your penis because unlike inserting malleable rod implants within your penis, it leaves your penis with a natural appearance. To add, contrary to penile prosthesis, if ever vascular reconstructive surgery is unsuccessful, it will not interfere with other treatments you are undergoing to cure erectile dysfunction.

However, it must be noted that not every man who is suffering from erectile dysfunction whose cause is organic can be candidates for vascular reconstructive surgery. Before you have the hopes of going through this kind of surgery, you have to submit yourself to a battery of extensive testing. And unfortunately, there is not a lot of medical centers around that have sufficient mastery and experience when it comes to vascular surgery for erectile dysfunction.

With all its advantages, it is understandable why this type of surgery is attractive. Unfortunately, aside from the fact that it is very expensive, its effectiveness is limited to only two years. Moreover, the surgery required for it is technically difficult which is precisely why only a few centers offer vascular reconstructive surgery services. There is also the risk of contracting an infection and experiencing numbness of your penis.

Vacuum pump therapy

In vacuum pump therapy, a man with ED will use a clear plastic cylinder where he will insert his penis into. He will then have to pump in order to force air out of the plastic cylinder, leaving a partial vacuum around the penis and facilitating the drawing of blood into the penis. The next step would be to put a special ring over the base of the shaft so that blood will be trapped inside it.

One clear advantage of vacuum pump therapy is it would not necessitate surgery. The only side downside to it is the bruising that you will experience from time to time if the vacuum is left on for too long.

Injection therapy

This kind of therapy involves the injection of a substance (i.e. drug) into the penis to help better flow of blood. The drug commonly used for this type of therapy and which the FDA has approved is called alprostadil. Alprostadil has the ability of relaxing muscle tissues, resulting to improved blood flow into the penis. Alprostadil is usually injected shortly before sexual intercourse.

The main concern with resorting to this type of therapy is the painful sensation of the injection process itself.

CONCLUSION

Now that you have reached the last part, I would like to thank you once again for downloading this book!

Having erectile dysfunction is hardly the end of the world. If your world revolves around your sex life, do not mourn for your penis because from what you learned in this book, there are ways to treat and overcome erectile dysfunction.

Erectile dysfunction has always been portrayed as one of the greatest nightmares for men and while it is true that it is a cause for concern, thinking that you are a failure as a man because of it is unwarranted and baseless. After all, erectile dysfunction is not permanent and there is so much you can do to get over this hurdle and live your sexual life the way you want to. So better erase those kinds of thoughts.

It is understandable why you, as the man, can feel devastated when you could not satisfy the needs of your partner. The negative emotions brought about by erectile dysfunction can trigger a cascade of events that could lead to couples distancing from each other both physically and emotionally. But always bear in mind that erectile dysfunction is just another medical condition. Just like how another kind of disease may render you unable to have sex for a period of time, erectile dysfunction works like that, too. You should not treat erectile dysfunction as something bigger and scarier that what it truly is. It is when you start to let ED define your identity and it is when you begin to measure your worth as a man to how successful you are in achieving and keeping an erection that the complications start to pile up.

For women reading this book, I hope by now that you have understood what your partner suffering through erectile dysfunction could be feeling during this whole predicament. When he detaches himself from you, do not assume that he is abandoning you or no longer feels that you are attractive. Practice open communication with your partner and realize that regardless of the type and severity, medical conditions could definitely affect a person in ways that you might not like.

Moreover, if your partner is not handling his condition well and is burying himself in his own head, take the responsibility of educating him and present him with his options. Make him understand that there is something that can be done. Encourage him to seek treatment as it can be a signal of any health condition such as those mentioned like the most common – diabetes.

For guys out there, in spite of what you are experiencing, your sexual and social life need not suffer too what with all the possible treatment methods we have discussed in this book. You can overcome erectile dysfunction and you will be ready and roaring in no time at all!

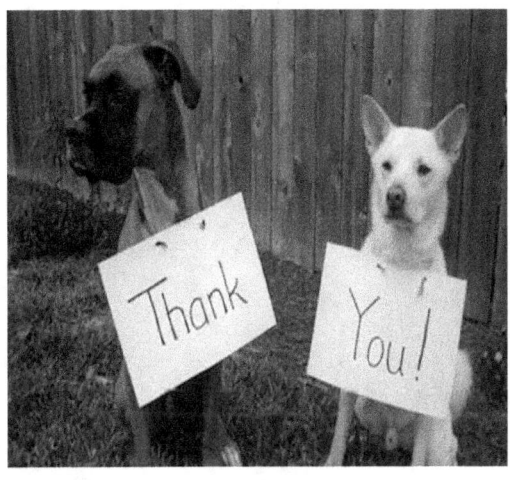

Finally, if you enjoyed this book, then I'd like to ask you for a favor, would you be kind enough to leave a review for this book on Amazon? It'd be greatly appreciated! Thank you and good luck!